RESTORE YOUR HEALTH WITH THE WISE GINSENG CHOICE

The powerful answer to:

- Lack of Energy, Fatigue, Exhaustion
- Cancer, Diabetes, Alzheimer's and more
- Sexual Performance

Terry Lemerond

and

Jacob Teitelbaum, M.D.

The purpose of this book is to educate. It is not intended to serve as a replacement for professional medical advice. Any use of the information in this book is at the reader's discretion. This book is sold with the understanding that neither the publisher nor the author has any liability or responsibility for any injury caused or alleged to be caused directly or indirectly by the information contained in this book. While every effort has been made to ensure its accuracy, the book's contents should not be construed as medical advice. To obtain medical advice on your individual health needs, please consult a qualified health care practitioner.

www.TTNPublishing.com

Library of Congress Control Number: 2023914675

Print ISBN: 978-1-952507-50-2
eBook ISBN: 978-1-952507-51-9

Editor: Michele Olson
Design: Kristy Frisque
Formatting: Alt 19 Creative

Printed in the United States of America

This book is dedicated to all the true health seekers in the world.

Contents

CHAPTER 1
A Prized Herbal Remedy

Ginseng. Or maybe we should say, "Ginseng!"

You've no doubt heard of ginseng. You've probably heard of its energy-giving superpowers and more. That's why we subconsciously add an exclamation mark when we think of ginseng and how much it contributes to human health and how much it is prized as an herbal remedy. It's that important in the plant world.

Health care practitioners in the know will prescribe ginseng if you're feeling the worn out, exhausted, stressed, foggy brained, can't sleep blues. In other words, you're the victim of the challenges and ills of the modern world. You're not alone!

Ginseng is certainly the energy herb. It's a tonic that banishes fatigue and ramps up your performance whether you're a marathoner or an evening stroll lover. Ginseng is proven to prolong life compared to those who don't take it. Add in ginseng's effectiveness against cognitive dysfunction, including brain fog, chronic fatigue syndrome, mental fatigue and, in its most severe form, Alzheimer's disease. In addition, extensive research shows that *Panax ginseng* is an effective treatment for cancer, diabetes, erectile dysfunction, and menopausal symptoms. It's a winner in anybody's book.

To give you an idea of how highly prized Panax ginseng is in Asian medicine, simply look at its name. Panax comes from the Greek word "panacea," which means "cure for all." Traditionally, it is valued as a miraculous plant, helping numerous other conditions including the above.

For example, it is considered both calming and energizing. Picture what it would feel like to have calm energy! It even has been valued as an aphrodisiac and antidepressant!

Those natural practitioners who love ginseng are right—in a way, but on the other hand, the ginseng on their shelves or at your local health food store might not be very helpful. Stay with us. We'll explain.

GINSENG, GINSENOSIDES, GINTONINS, WHAT??

Let's just step back for a moment and take a look at this Asian medicinal powerhouse herb that has been used in traditional Chinese medicine (TCM) and other Eastern and Western natural healing traditions for thousands of years.

There are nearly a dozen varieties of ginseng, but the two best known and most commonly used medicinals are *Panax ginseng* (better known as red ginseng or Asian or Korean ginseng) and American ginseng, *Panax quinquefolius.* The two plants have varying uses, as does Siberian ginseng, which is not part of the Panax family and has totally different benefits. American ginseng is often used for its relaxant and calmative properties and Asian ginseng is prized for its invigorating effects and more, as you'll learn in this book.

Ginseng's medicinal qualities are found in its fleshy root that is uniquely shaped like a human body. Healers have long believed that ginseng embodies three mythical essences of humans—body, mind, and spirit.

AN HERB BY MANY NAMES

Panax ginseng is most often called red ginseng and sometimes called Asian or Korean ginseng.

Normally, *Panax ginseng* is a slow-growing root that takes about twenty years to mature in the wild. But Belgian researchers have recently discovered a process that accelerates the growth cycle while carefully cultivating the plants during every stage of production for stable and certified quality. This process also enhances the availability of certain healing compounds to your body. Stay with us.

Within these varieties of ginseng, there are types of *Panax ginseng* that contain varying types and amounts of the active chemical compounds called ginsenosides.

Let's start with white and red ginseng. They are from *Panax ginseng,* but they are processed differently. White ginseng is made from a peeled root and red ginseng is made from the whole root, steamed and dried to a characteristic red color. Red and white ginsengs have varying uses, but red ginseng is widely considered the most effective remedy for a wide variety of health issues.

But let's go a little farther.

Ginsenosides, also known as steroid-like saponins, are only found in the ginseng family and are responsible for many of the herb's healing qualities. Ginsenosides are, of course, contained in both red and white ginseng, but there are far more ginsenosides in red ginseng. Some of the most important have names that sound more like alphabet soup: Rb1 and Rb2 fight inflammation, Rd and Re that neutralize disease-causing free radicals and protect nerve cells, Rp1, Rg3 and Rh2 that attack cancer in a variety of ways and Rg1 that addresses the underlying causes of Alzheimer's disease and dozens more.

These major ginsenosides can be converted into rare ginsenosides by microorganisms in the digestive tract, making them far more potent healing agents and more available for your body to use (bioavailable).

Rare ginsenosides (sometimes called noble ginsenosides) amp up the healing powers of the ginseng plant, especially when it is grown and processed in a particular way.

Among many other healing benefits, rare ginsenosides have been found to have potent anti-cancer effects, especially against lung cancer. We'll go into this more in Chapter 5.

Plus a multitude of other beneficial nutrients are found in red ginseng, including phenols, polysaccharides, lignans, amino acids, minerals and more, each making a unique contribution to the healing powers of ginseng.

In addition, red ginseng belongs to an elite class of herbs called adaptogens. It's at the top of the list that includes such health powerhouses as *Rhodiola rosea, Andrographis paniculata, Eleutherococcus senticosus (Siberian ginseng)* and *Schizandra chinensis.*

We'll go into the subject of adaptogens in depth in Chapter 3, but for now, it's important to know that this elite class of plant medicines give your body what it needs to survive and thrive. It also acts as a "vaccine" against mental stress and the myriad ways it can negatively affect your health.

This amazingly complex series of synergistic interactions of molecular networks and cellular communication systems quite literally offers your body healing power that adds up to more than the sum of the parts.

HAVING AN ENERGY CRISIS?

Soooo—Have you ever said anything like this about yourself?

"I feel like an old dish rag."

"I just can't get out of bed in the morning"

"I'm useless without my morning coffee."

"I need more coffee to make it through my day."

"I wish I had my 30-year-old body back."

There are two basic types of fatigue—short-term fatigue, like the kind you experience after a good workout or a long run. Then there's long-term or chronic fatigue. Short-term fatigue disappears after a good rest and a drink of water. Chronic fatigue never seems to go away, no matter how much you rest, and it often gets worse with time.

Then it becomes a vicious circle: You're tired, so you use stimulants, like caffeine, to pick up your energy, which it does, for an hour or two. But then caffeine disrupts your sleep cycles, leaving you more and more tired, spiraling down into profound exhaustion that messes with your memory, your ability to concentrate, and your work productivity. It seems like there's no way out of that hole.

Bottom line? You want to increase energy wisely, using herbs and nutrients that create healthy energy instead of acting like energy loan sharks!

WHY NOT BUY MY GINSENG AT THE DRUG STORE?

Here's the rub: Most ginseng on the market has limited bioavailability. That means that even though the healing power is there, our bodies can't use it well, so ginseng's effect is minimal. Much of the ginseng on today's market is heavily sprayed with pesticides, which get concentrated into the roots of the plant. It becomes even more concentrated when the plants are steamed, dried and powdered, and inserted into capsules for the consumer market. Do you really want to put that into your body?

Most of the ginsenosides are poorly absorbed in the intestine, so they are not readily available (bioavailable) for your body to use. Scientists have discovered that many ginsenosides are destroyed as they pass through the digestive tract and, in most supplements, the ginsenosides' potency was too short-lived to have the desired effects.

In fact, most conventionally processed ginseng (which by the way, is often processed using toxic solvents) releases as little as 20% of those potent ginsenosides and rare ginsenosides.

WHAT IF . . .?

What if we told you that there is a process that uses a 100% natural cultivation method, producing a pure whole ginseng containing eight of the most important ginsenosides, with a potency five- to ten-fold higher and far more bioavailable than traditionally processed brands?

The good news? It's true. There is such a process.

Wild ginseng has been overharvested and is increasingly hard to find. Therefore, providers have moved to farming. Since farmed ginseng is quite vulnerable to pests, it is sprayed with huge amounts of toxic pesticides and herbicides to create a commercially viable crop.

A new aquaculture method renders all that obsolete. There is no spraying whatsoever. The scientists created a complex nutrient system to maximize the bioavailability of the ginsenosides in the roots. However, for ginseng to be powerful, you can't just feed it what it needs to thrive. You must strategically stress the plant for the ginsenosides to fully develop. But you can't stress it so much that it causes permanent damage. It's a tricky and very specific process.

This cutting-edge hydroponic red ginseng growing method has been scientifically validated to produce ginseng that is more powerful and more bioavailable than any product now on the market.

Scientific assays show this ginseng is 17 times more absorbable and has seven times the levels of rare ginsenosides as standard ginseng. It has an equivalent in ginsenoside profile to 20-year old wild ginseng.

This novel method of growing red ginseng is possible thanks to groundbreaking technology that simulates a "perfect spring" by regulating the growing temperature and by simulating stressors like insect attacks to increase the plants' anti-stress healing power.

Additionally, this ginseng is produced without the use of any pesticides or herbicides. The vertical farming technique is not only environmentally sustainable, it is completely in line with environmental responsibility.

Once harvested, the hydroponically-grown ginseng undergoes traditional Korean steam processing that respects the plant and naturally fosters a wonderfully high content of rare ginsenosides. It's the perfect marriage of new and old—and the ultimate beneficiary is you!

Ready to add one of the most revered and powerful Asian herbal remedies to your healthcare toolkit? This is the biggest thing to hit the ginseng market in a very, very long time.

WHAT YOU NEED TO KNOW:

- *Panax ginseng* has for centuries been revered as a healing and energizing tonic, especially to combat fatigue.
- It has now been scientifically confirmed as effective against a host of diseases, including cancer, Alzheimer's, diabetes and more.
- Active compounds in ginsenosides and rare ginsenosides not only help boost energy and banish chronic fatigue, but also provide important tools to combat the underlying causes of diseases.
- *Panax ginseng* (steamed and dried) is also commonly known as red ginseng or Korean ginseng.
- A new ginseng cultivation method concentrates the medicinal compounds in ginseng, makes them more usable by your body and shortens the growing time while being completely environmentally responsible and sustainable.

CHAPTER 2
The Great Multi-Tasker

Panax ginseng has a bit of everything you need for a long, healthy life.

You've probably heard the word "synergy." It means something is greater than the sum of its parts. It's a perfect word to describe red ginseng and the three powerful healing properties that attack health problems, especially the diseases most commonly associated with aging, and bring your body back into balance:

Adaptogen
Anti-inflammatory
Antioxidant

When you bring those three powerhouses together, ginseng's abilities are remarkable when it comes to restoring youthful vitality and overcoming the deterioration most of us associate with aging.

Let's take them one at a time:

ADAPTOGEN

At the top of the triad, ginseng's value is that it is an adaptogen. You may not be familiar with the word, but adaptogens are the multi-taskers of the plant world. In the simplest possible terms, adaptogens like ginseng and a handful of others are plant medicines that provide your body what it needs to survive and thrive.

Adaptogen have the potential to provide plant-based treatments for a wide variety of diseases, chronic conditions, and syndromes. This is an amazingly complex series of synergistic interactions of molecular networks and cellular communication systems that quite literally add up to more than the sum of the parts.

Adaptogens play a key role defending your body against environmental challenges, including harmful bacteria, diseases carried by insects (think of ticks and Lyme disease, mosquitoes and malaria), excessive ultraviolet rays from the sun and challenges from pollution, temperature fluctuations and more.

The key to understanding adaptogens is that they help establish and maintain homeostasis, the body's internal wisdom that brings all systems into balance. It does this by building your natural resistance to stressors—physical, chemical, biological, and psychological.

Adaptogens like ginseng actually work like healthy stress vaccines to activate your body's defense and stress response systems and metabolic rate. They reverse the negative physical effects of stress and restore your body to balance and health.

If your immune system is not functioning properly by overreacting or underreacting to challenges, ginseng supports the correct immune response.

If your immune system is overly active, triggering allergies and asthma or rheumatoid arthritis or lupus and other autoimmune diseases, ginseng will lower the immune system's response and return it to a normal level.

If your immune system is underactive, and you frequently get colds, bronchitis, sinus or ear infections and even pneumonia, or you have anemia or digestive problems like ulcers or chronic diarrhea, ginseng can help strengthen your immune response and break the cycle of illness.

If your brain chemistry is unbalanced, ginseng can return it to balance, having profound effects on cognitive function, memory and mood, as you'll see in the coming chapters.

The power of adaptogens goes far beyond the immune system.

Adaptogens like ginseng can correct imbalances in cellular division cycles that cause cells to divide wildly, eventually causing cancer.

Many people use adaptogens to prevent or postpone the chronic diseases of aging, recognizing their uncanny ability to fix what's wrong, boost what's right, keep your body in balance and prevent body functions from deteriorating.

Adaptogenic powers like those we see in ginseng have been scientifically validated as effective against chronic inflammation, atherosclerosis (hardening of the arteries), neurodegenerative cognitive impairment (Alzheimer's disease and other forms of dementia), metabolic disorders, diabetes, cancer and a host of other age-related diseases.

INFLAMMATION

What happens when you hit your thumb with a hammer or twist an ankle or bonk your head? Of course, it hurts! Within minutes, the site of the injury becomes red, swells and may feel hot. You may limp on that twisted ankle or even be unable to walk on it at all.

Acute—meaning short-term—inflammation is the result of an injury of some sort. "Short-term" is the key—the swelling and heat awaken your body's natural healing mechanisms. The injury heals, and you go on with your life.

Acute inflammation is a good thing. The swelling protects the healing tissues, clears out damaged tissues, starts the healing process and the pain reminds you to be gentle with the injured area.

But there is another type of inflammation that is much less obvious and much more dangerous: Long-term inflammation may have no clear symptoms, yet it is an underlying cause of a host of life-threatening diseases.

Inflammation is the immune system's response when it's challenged. We need inflammation when we have an injury or other challenge. Yet there are times when we don't need inflammation and when it can be incredibly destructive.

That's right—it's systemic or chronic inflammation that science has proven is behind heart disease, cancer, type 2 diabetes, obesity, Alzheimer's disease, chronic obstructive pulmonary disorder (COPD), inflammatory bowel disease, and many more diseases of aging.

If that's not bad enough, inflammation is also an underlying factor in allergies and autoimmune diseases like lupus, type 1 diabetes, rheumatoid arthritis, and celiac disease.

And then, there is arthritis, the obvious inflammatory disease that manifests as swelling and pain, but unlike acute inflammation, the pain and swelling don't go away. Many types of arthritis may start with an injury, for example a knee or shoulder injury that never really heals, and over time, shifts from acute inflammation to chronic inflammation, eventually causing the cushioning joint tissues to deteriorate.

Chronic inflammation, where this important repair system goes out of balance, is a major contributor to most health problems affecting most people.

It goes without saying that you want to knock out chronic inflammation. And here comes red ginseng—the excess inflammation slayer. One impressive Korean animal study published in 2018 in the *Journal of Ginseng Research* showed that 11 ginsenosides in *Panax ginseng* reduced lung inflammation by more than half in some subjects, showing it was at least as effective as dexamethasone, a steroid drug widely used to treat chronic obstructive pulmonary disease (COPD), asthma, and other serious lung diseases.

Chinese researchers have credited the ginsenoside Rg1 with substantial reduction in swelling and pain in animals with arthritis.

Other research confirms red ginseng's effectiveness against the inflammation that is an underlying cause of type 2 diabetes, cancer, gastrointestinal disorders, arthritis, and hepatitis.

ANTIOXIDANT

We need oxygen to live, so how can oxidation be a bad thing? Because high levels of oxygen in your body can be corrosive and toxic.

Think of rust on the bumper of your car—scientifically it's caused by unstable oxygen molecules that are missing an electron or two. Along the same lines, unstable oxygen molecules, called free radicals, cause "rust" on your cells, damaging DNA. It also disrupts cellular reproduction, so new cells are not exact copies of the parent cells. This is how aging cells open the way to diseases caused by imperfect cell reproduction and growth.

Our bodies are bombarded by free radicals 24/7. Toxins in air, food, water, cigarette smoke, industrial pollutants, pesticides, herbicides, and other environmental toxins contribute to the free radical population explosion, sometimes called oxidative stress.

Yet, we are not helpless against this onslaught. Antioxidants found in plant foods and nutrients stop free radicals by donating electrons to help stabilize these electrically challenged oxygen molecules and neutralize their destructive potential.

Antioxidants like those found in red ginseng are among the most powerful forces in the plant world against free radical damage and the diseases of aging.

In fact, in an animal study, Korean researchers found that the antioxidants in red ginseng extract reversed free radical damage and restored youthful vitality in aging animals. Centuries of experience show that the same is true for humans.

IN CONCLUSION . . .

Remember we said that the ginsenosides in red ginseng combine to provide a synergistic weapon against disease that strikes the disease process from several directions, each unique component increasing the healing powers of the others?

Now you probably understand why.

The power of red ginseng is abundantly clear. Its unique ability to restore balance to all the body's systems as an adaptogen, its power against inflammation, the underlying cause of many of the most serious diseases of aging. Its antioxidant effect makes red ginseng the most important tool in anyone's anti-aging toolkit.

WHAT YOU NEED TO KNOW:

Red ginseng prevents serious disease conditions in three primary ways.

It's:

- A proven adaptogen that restores balance to stressed body systems
- An anti-inflammatory that reverses body-destroying inflammation, the underlying cause of many diseases, as well as aging; and
- An antioxidant that neutralizes disease-causing free radical oxygen molecules.

CHAPTER 3
Curcumin: Where's My Get Up and Go?

If you're feeling overwhelmed, exhausted, or generally drained, if your "get up and go" got up and went, you're not alone.

According to the National Institutes of Health, severe fatigue affects one in every five Americans. Other research suggests that 31% of American adults suffer from exhaustion. As many as 4% have the worst forms of the human energy crisis, chronic fatigue syndrome and fibromyalgia. A recent survey by the National Safety Council found that nearly half of us—43%—say we are too tired to function well at work.

Worse yet, one in 25 drivers over 18 admitted they have fallen asleep at the wheel in the last month. The National Highway Traffic Safety Administration estimates that drowsy driving caused 72,000 crashes, 6,000 of them fatal. The National Safety Council says a person who has lost two hours of sleep from a normal eight-hour sleep schedule could be as impaired as a person who has consumed up to three beers.

The bottom line? Who do you know who wouldn't love more energy? Wouldn't you?

The unrelenting stress of the modern lifestyle is at the heart of much of our fatigue and feelings of being overwhelmed. Information overload, back-to-back commitments, long commutes, the needs of kids and spouses, and long work hours can leave you physically and mentally drained. Meanwhile, the news media seems to feel that it should turn everything into a crisis and that everybody should hate each other. Add in the physiological stressors of air pollution, chemical contamination of our food, general poor diets, and the constant presence of technology, and you get the picture.

Have you ever said your brain is tired? Mental fatigue is just one more of the results of our hectic lifestyles. You're probably rolling your eyes right now and saying, "Welcome to my life."

Fatigue is a complex medical issue that even the experts have difficulty understanding, much less explaining or treating. It becomes even more complex because it manifests in different ways in different individuals.

Besides the obvious effects on your ability to function physically, being chronically exhausted can lead to adrenal fatigue and even adrenal exhaustion. The adrenals, those two tiny glands that sit on top of your kidneys, produce a variety of hormones, including the stress hormone cortisol. When you are constantly in a state of stress, it's like constantly having the gas pedal to the metal. Eventually, you'll run out of gas and you might even blow your engine.

The simplest way to tell if you have adrenal exhaustion? Do you get irritable when hungry? This has been called being "Hangry"! The worst thing you can do when this happens is eat sugar or a candy bar. Instead, you need to support your exhausted adrenal glands.

Continually pushing yourself past your limits can lead to serious health consequences. Chronic stress can also impair your memory and concentration. It can also lead to weight gain and a weakened immune system, leaving you less able to fight off disease.

If you're not taking time to recharge, you're probably sinking deeper and deeper into exhaustion and maybe even depression. Whether you've been burning the candle at both ends lately or running on fumes for as long as you can remember, adding the most bioavailable form of ginseng to your daily routine will lift your lagging energy levels.

THE ENERGIZER BUNNY

Anyone with even a modest knowledge of herb lore can probably tell you that ginseng is the energy herb.

Our ancient ancestors called it a tonic, and modern science credits the adaptogenic effects of Korean ginseng for the energy it provides in the short and long term.

A study published in 2007 confirms that red ginseng helped reduce levels of the stress hormone cortisol when lab animals were subjected to stressful situations. This means ginseng taken daily can keep us on an even keel and stop the stress cycle from spiraling out of control and prevent adrenal fatigue.

A growing number of studies point to red ginseng as a safe and effective way to reduce mental and physical fatigue and restore vitality.

One 2016 review published in the *Journal of Korean Medical Science* took a deep look at 12 randomized clinical trials involving 630 people and found that those taking a ginseng supplement experienced a marked reduction of their fatigue.

Another randomized study in the *Journal of Ginseng Research* reported that, among patients with fatty liver disease experiencing fatigue, red ginseng helped to restore energy levels, especially in the participants who were also overweight.

And another six-week trial of 63 subjects living a high stress lifestyle added even more evidence to Korean red ginseng's energizing effects. This study, which also appeared in the *Journal of Ginseng Research,* randomized the participants to either a red ginseng supplement or a placebo. At the end of the study, those in the ginseng group reported less mental stress and improved mood. Testing revealed that the red ginseng appeared to ease mental fatigue by stabilizing the sympathetic nervous system. The researchers also noted improved brain function in those taking the herb.

Red ginseng is so powerful that it has even been shown to be helpful in those with chronic fatigue syndrome. Among 90 patients with idiopathic chronic fatigue syndrome (which means that doctors couldn't pinpoint an underlying cause), those taking the herb found relief from their unrelenting fatigue. The researchers speculated that ginseng's antioxidant activity—which can be attributed to the ginsenosides in the herb—were at least partially responsible for its energizing effects.

An interesting Brazilian study found that women diagnosed with fibromyalgia were able to reduce their pain levels by 39.4% and their fatigue levels by 46.5% in just six weeks, similar to the symptom reduction in those who took amitriptyline, a pharmaceutical with numerous common side effects including drowsiness, dizziness, weight gain, and increased hunger. The study participants who took red ginseng had no serious side effects.

Interestingly, ginseng works by shutting down overactivity of pain molecules called NMDA. This plays an especially important role in fibromyalgia, and the very few medications that settle down NMDA can have severe toxicities. This makes ginseng a potentially very remarkable tool for pain relief, especially for those with chronic pain.

Depression and anxiety commonly accompany chronic stress. We'll go into this in greater detail in Chapter 4, but depression leads to brain cell dysfunction, so it's important to stop depression at the earliest levels possible. Chinese researchers found that red ginseng was at least as effective as fluoxetine (Prozac) in treating depression and anxiety.

Studies also confirm that elevated stress levels lead to more pain and ultimately to spiraling levels of stress and anxiety. It is clear from this body of research that breaking the cycle of stress, anxiety, and depression has positive effects on all the mechanisms of the human body.

It's important to point out here that almost all of the studies mentioned in this book were carried out on *Panax ginseng* formulated in the conventional way, not with the significantly more powerful hydroponic red ginseng formulation. We think it's reasonable to conclude that the positive effects would be even greater when more of the active ginsenosides and rare ginsenosides are available for the human body to use.

SIDE EFFECTS

Red ginseng is safe and effective if taken at recommended daily dosages of .5 to 2 g of dried root.

The only documented side effect is a reduction of blood glucose content due to ginseng's ability to control blood sugar. If you are taking diabetes drugs, you should consult your doctor before taking it.

The herb has not been evaluated for pregnant women or nursing moms, so it's best to avoid it at those times.

WHAT YOU NEED TO KNOW:

Red ginseng has been used as an energy tonic for at least 3,000 years and it's best known for those healing benefits. It has been scientifically proven to:

- Stop the serious health effects of long-term chronic stress by reducing levels of the stress hormone, cortisol
- Relieve fatigue and exhaustion that commonly result from the chronic stress
- Relieve anxiety and depression as well as commonly used pharmaceuticals without serious side effects

CHAPTER 4
A Better Brain

Ginseng's almost magical abilities to boost energy are even greater when we start looking into brain function.

It stands to reason that ginsenosides can address mental fatigue as well as physical fatigue-and science validates this. But new research takes the issue several steps farther.

MEMORY LOSS AND AGING

Memory loss is one of the greatest challenges of Western society.

Memory loss that is associated with the normal process of aging, sometimes called Age Related Cognitive Decline (ARCD), is far different from Alzheimer's disease and other forms of dementia. Slow reaction times, slower abilities to recall information, longer time required to complete a task, and diminished abilities to multi-task are frequently cited as characteristics of ARCD.

Some of us think that we grow less mentally sharp as we age. We think much—maybe most—of this type of cognitive decline is a self-fulfilling prophecy. We *think* we slow down as we age, and so we do. Most of us can be as mentally astute as we have always been—provided we get proper diet, exercise and mental stimulation.

ALZHEIMER'S AND DEMENTIA

Alzheimer's disease, the most serious form of dementia, slowly damages brain cells. The cause is not known and there are few, if any, useful treatments.

The incidence of Alzheimer's is steadily increasing. As of this writing, 5.5 million Americans have been diagnosed with the disease, most of them over 65. Two-thirds of them are women. Those numbers are expected to increase to 13.8 million by 2050.

This brings into play the relatively new science of neurogenesis. Until very recently, scientists believed that we were born with all the neurons we would ever have in our lifetimes, so if we lost neurons (brain cells), we would lose brain function. It was believed that Alzheimer's and other forms of dementia were caused by a shortage of neurons. That didn't make sense even back in the days before neurogenesis was affirmed in the late 1990s, since all cells in the human body die and regenerate themselves constantly, and it wouldn't even be logical to think that brain cells were somehow excluded from the law of apoptosis or programmed cell death.

Of course, it turns out that brain cells are born and die throughout our lifetimes like all other cells.

Remember those nutrient powerhouses called ginsenosides? These nutrients are key to the impressive healing qualities of this.

Now scientists have found another ginsenoside, Compound K, an active end metabolite, which means it is a byproduct of the breakdown of other ginsenosides (in this case Rb1, Rb2 and Rc), detected in blood and urine tests.

Compound K and other rare ginsenosides (Rg5, Rk1, Rg3 and Rg6) have well-recognized effects to improve memory, to protect the brain from age-related cognitive decline, and to decrease the effects of Alzheimer's disease and cerebral ischemia (reduced blood flow to the brain that can lead to a stroke).

Compound K is a known antioxidant, so neutralizing the free radical oxygen molecules in the brain may account for some of the ginsenoside's effects.

In 2009, scientists identified the potential of ginsenosides Rg5, Rk1 and Rg3 to be used for treatment of neurodegenerative diseases like Alzheimer's where memory loss is connected to the loss of neurons, the brain cells that carry information. This study shows that Rg3 and Rg5 protect neurons in case of physiological stress.

Moreover, lab studies also showed that Rg3 can enhance memory by decreasing microglial activation (a hallmark of brain diseases), lowering inflammation and restores normal cell life spans, all of which are present in neurodegenerative conditions.

A review from 2018 reported two main active ingredients of ginseng that produce anti-Alzheimer's effects: rare ginsenosides, like Rh2, and the lysophosphatidic acids (LPAs) present in gintonin. Animal studies showed that both protect against the formation of beta-amyloid plaque typical of Alzheimer's and reinforce the brain cholinergic systems that regulate attention and complex cognitive function.

Moreover, rare ginsenosides decreased oxidative stress, while gintonin increased the creation of new cells in the hippocampus, the memory center of the brain.

The authors of the Korean study concluded, "The plethora of potential health benefits of rare ginsenosides like compound K, Rg3, Rg5, Rg6, and Rh2, warrants further research to evaluate its biochemical mechanisms and its ability to protect healthy populations from neurodegenerative diseases."

An Austrian review concludes that Compound K and other ginsenosides prevent neurons from dying prematurely, counteracting environmental toxins, the release of free radicals and rises in intercellular calcium, overstimulation by the neurotransmitter glutamate and the interruption of the normal cellular life cycle. The Austrian authors concluded, ". . . neuroprotective actions of ginsenosides could come about as a valuable option to slow down neurodegenerative diseases."

A broad Korean study of nearly 4,000 elders concluded that long-term use of ginseng resulted in better memory as they entered their later years. Knowing that the use of ginseng as a general tonic and energy producer is part of several Asian cultures, it's good to know that the earlier you start using *Panax ginseng*, the better.

However, other studies show that short courses of *Panax ginseng* can also have profound effects, although there are some mixed opinions that echo the conclusion of the Korean study that more research is warranted.

MENTAL CLARITY

Of course, brain issues go far beyond memory. Some simple ones are the ability to concentrate and perform well on testing at any age.

Human studies show that red ginseng can have a beneficial impact on cognition, as well as your memory and your mood.

In one small clinical trial published in the *Journal of Ginseng Research*, researchers found that those participants of varying ages who took a high-dose *Panax ginseng* supplement scored significantly better on cognition tests than those taking a placebo.

Another eight-day study found that a daily dose of red ginseng increased feelings of calmness while also improving math skills.

Scientists speculate that these improvements are a result of the herb's ginsenoside content and its ability to protect the brain against damaging free radicals.

An interesting British study also suggests that Compound K improves the brain's transmission system. It works like this: Neurons are brain cells. Dendrites are thread-like appendages to the neurons that work like an electrical system and pass on messages between neurons. If that transmission system is interrupted, the messages—whether they are thoughts, hormone signals or something else—don't get through or they are garbled. When Compound K improves the communication system or protects it from being damaged, memory is preserved.

DEPRESSION AND ANXIETY

Ginseng's ability to reduce stress is key to its ability to help people suffering from depression and anxiety. Long-term depression is closely linked to memory loss because it damages nerve cells. Nerve cell damage plus inflammation in the brain interrupts the process of neurogenesis, robbing the hippocampus, the brain's memory storage system, of the cells it needs to store and access memory.

Depression and anxiety frequently occur together. Preliminary animal research suggests that ginsenosides reduce anxiety. Studies have shown red ginseng is as effective a fluoxetine (Prozac), a pharmaceutical anti-anxiety drug that has numerous serious side effects.

As one of its many potent benefits, ginseng has been shown to help rebalance the major stress system in the body, called the hypothalamic-pituitary-adrenal axis.

It's also known that people with depression and anxiety are prone to other types of illness that may seem to be unrelated. It's not yet clear which is the cart, and which is the horse: Does the pain of diseases like cancer, heart disease, osteoporosis, and rheumatoid arthritis trigger depression and anxiety or do depression and anxiety predispose us to those diseases? Science hasn't given us an answer yet, but since we know for sure that *Panax ginseng* is a powerful tool against all of these illnesses, it should be a primary tool in nearly everyone's medicine chest.

WHAT YOU NEED TO KNOW:

Red ginseng has been scientifically validated to:

- Protect brain cells from damage due to environmental toxins
- Prevent brain cells from early or premature death
- Improve mental clarity
- Improve memory
- Improve performance on tests
- Improve energy while reducing anxiety and depression
- Be as effective as some prescription drugs to ease depression and anxiety without serious side effects.

CHAPTER 5
Cancer Combatant

Cancer is a terrible disease that modern medicine has yet to conquer.

Despite billions upon billions of dollars spent on research, billions spent on healthcare and an untold toll in human lives, the cure eludes us. Current knowledge suggests that every cancer is bio-individual—scientific language for everyone is different and all cancers are different.

Yet, of course, there are some common threads.

Most cancers:

- Create a network of blood vessels to sustain and nourish cancerous cells
- Are the result of the failure of the system that governs the natural life spans and reproduction of all cells
- May spread to other body systems

THE DISEASE WITH MANY FACES

Most of us know someone who has cancer and, sadly, many of us know someone who has died of cancer.

The National Cancer Institute reports that 1,735,350 new cases of cancer were diagnosed in 2018 and 609,640 people died of the disease.

The most common types of cancer in the U.S. are (in descending order, according to estimated new cases in 2018):

- breast
- lung and bronchial
- prostate
- colorectal
- melanoma
- bladder
- non-Hodgkin's lymphoma
- kidney and renal
- endometrial
- leukemia
- pancreatic
- thyroid
- liver

FOUR MEANS OF ATTACK

Remember back in Chapter 1, we mentioned that white ginseng is steam processed to become red ginseng?

It turns out that *Panax ginseng* has powerful anti-cancer properties that University of Chicago researchers say originate in the steaming process that transforms raw ginseng into red ginseng.

Their 2016 study published in the *Chinese Journal of Natural Medicine* confirms that the steaming process transforms certain tongue-twisting ginsenosides, called protopanaxadiols and protopanaxatriols, into formidable cancer-fighting rare ginsenosides.

The superpowers generated during the steam process mean that red ginseng (Korean ginseng) fights cancer in four important ways:

- Apoptosis
- Cell cycle arrest
- Angiogenesis
- Anti-metastatic

Let's take a look at each one:

APOPTOSIS AND CELL CYCLE ARREST

We're putting these together because they are closely related, but different.

As we are sure you know from high school biology, all cells in the human body have a specific life span, programmed into our DNA. Our cells are living and dying every single minute of our lives and each cell is programmed to adhere to a finite life span.

Sometimes the cells' messages to reproduce get garbled and some inner intelligence knows the new cells won't be an exact copy of the old ones, so it stops the process of cell division.

Other times, the message doesn't get through and cells fail to die at the end of their natural life span, a biological process called apoptosis. In a strange sequence, chemical messages are sent to the cells, telling them quite literally to commit suicide. The DNA of the cells is destroyed by enzymes released because of these chemical messages, the cell's surface bubbles away and chemical sweepers usher the dead cells out of the body.

Healthy red blood cells live for about four months and they are replaced with new healthy cells. White blood cells live for a year or more, but skin cells live only two or three weeks; colon cells die after about only four days. The human body replaces an astonishing one million cells per second.

Sometimes things go wrong for reasons not yet fully understood by modern science, when apoptosis fails, and cells don't die at the end of their normal life span. With cancer, those immortal cells can continue indefinitely, clump together to form tumors and can eventually kill the patient.

Chinese research confirms that the Rg3 ginsenoside in Korean ginseng restores the natural process of apoptosis in human oral cancer cells and another Chinese study found similar effects of Rg3 against liver cancer cells.

A 2018 Korean study confirmed that *Panax ginseng* stopped the cycle that formed lung cancer cells, further validated by Chinese research on colorectal cancer cells.

ANGIOGENESIS

All living things need nourishment in some form. Cancer cells are no exception. As a cancerous tumor begins to form, it will also develop a network of blood vessels to provide nutrients and oxygen, so the tumor can grow and thrive. Cancers, driven by their hunger for survival, find ways to obtain what they need by creating their own system of blood vessels designed specifically to deliver nutrients and oxygen.

This process, called angiogenesis, helps ensure the survival of the cancer cells, and the disease.

In the *Journal of Ginseng Rese*arch, a 2017 study shows that red ginseng's Rg1 and Rb1 ginsenosides marshal a group of small, but powerful, cancer fighting genes called microRNAs.

You may remember from biology class that RNA carries genetic information. The microRNAs are a form of RNA that can control hundreds, maybe thousands of genes and tell the body to stop producing blood vessels to feed cancerous tumors.

Another study published at the same time by University of Chicago researchers confirms the microRNA action and adds that certain ginsenosides may also contribute to cutting off the oxygen supply to the tumor-feeding blood vessels.

METASTASIS

Cancers want to hedge their bets. Not only are those cells capable of feeding themselves, they are also capable of entering the bloodstream and lymphatic system and spreading far and wide in the human body, the process called metastasis.

Cancer cells, like all cells, need glucose for survival. Not only that, cancer cells are slightly different from healthy cells. They are particularly dependent on glucose for survival, growth and metastasis. In fact, cancer cells thrive on sugar and they can trigger sugar cravings in their insatiable effort to survive. Table sugar (sucrose) is a particular favorite of cancer cells.

Cancer is an extremely complex disease. It's not as simple as saying eliminating sugar from your diet will stop the growth of cancer. It is fair to say that sugar is not healthy for anyone, so stopping eating sugar and fighting the sugar cravings that the cancer cells send out will certainly have an effect on your cancer risk as well as on the growth of some types of cancerous tumors.

Metastasis is the spread of cancer from its origin, known as the primary cancer site, to another part of the body. While metastasis is not an automatic death sentence, it will become one if it is not stopped.

Red ginseng has that base covered, too. Numerous studies show that ginsenosides are an effective way of stopping the spread of cancers. Among them, a 2011 Korean study showing that it stopped the migration of colon cancer cells to the lungs of laboratory animals. In 2012, Taiwanese researchers confirmed Korean ginseng's effectiveness in stopping liver cancer metastasis and a 2015 Korean study that found the same effect in arresting metastasis of melanoma skin cancer cells to the lungs.

OTHER WAYS IT WORKS . . .

Ginseng's anti-inflammatory effects help get at the root of a wide variety of cancers.

There has long been a folk myth that stress causes cancer. While stress may not directly cause cancer, the inflammation caused by unrelieved long-term stress is known to promote several diseases, including cancer.

Red ginseng has been shown to activate T and B cells, specialized defender cells that activate a strong immune system response and kill cancer cells (and attack other invaders as well).

CHEMO-ENHANCER

There is some evidence that Korean ginseng can enhance the effects of conventional chemotherapy and at least two studies show it helps protect healthy organs from damage by chemotherapy drugs.

PREVENTION

Red ginseng may even *prevent* certain types of cancer. A Korean study published in 2001 showed that people who used Korean ginseng had a 56% lower rate of all types of cancers compared to those who did not. Specifically, the greatest benefit was in prevention of lip, oral cavity, pharynx, esophageal, stomach, colorectal, liver, pancreatic, larynx, lung and ovarian cancers.

The authors wrote, "In conclusion, *Panax ginseng* has been established as non-organ specific cancer preventive, having dose response relationship. These results warrant that ginseng extracts and its synthetic derivatives should be examined for their preventive effect on various types of human cancers."

WHAT YOU NEED TO KNOW:

Ginseng is a powerful weapon against several types of cancer. It has been shown to be effective against some of the deadliest cancers, including melanoma, lung, liver, oral, pancreatic and colorectal cancers.

It has been shown to combat cancer in four specific ways:

- Tells cells to die at the end of their natural life span instead of converting into cancer
- Stops the blood vessel supply to tumors, effectively killing them
- Stops cancers from spreading
- Prevent cancers from starting in the first place

CHAPTER 6
Diabetes—Two Types—and Better Control

Diabetes is one of those sneaky diseases that causes its own problems and triggers a bunch of these down the road, any of which can be fatal.

Let's take a moment here for some simple biology: Your pancreas produces insulin, a hormone that regulates the amount of glucose or sugar in your blood.

There are two basic kinds of diabetes: type 1 and type 2. In the simplest possible terms, type 1 diabetes is characterized by the inability of the pancreas to produce insulin to balance blood sugar. People with type 2 diabetes are capable of producing insulin, but their bodies cannot use it. They are insulin resistant.

Both are terrible diseases that kill hundreds of thousands of Americans every year.

The good news—no, it's great news—is that red ginseng works wonderfully well against both types of diabetes.

Here's how:

GINSENG AND TYPE 1

Type 1 diabetes, most often diagnosed in children or young adults, is an autoimmune disease that attacks the cells in the pancreas that produce insulin.

Those who have the disease must take insulin injections to stay alive. Oral medications do not work for this type of diabetes. There are some nasty side effects when blood sugars aren't well controlled, including heart disease, epilepsy, thyroid disease, chronic lung disease, mental illness, colitis, gastritis, anemia, migraines, and an increased risk of cancer.

Most people with type 1 diabetes have some minimal pancreatic function, insulin production and release. It's just not enough to balance blood sugars.

Most conventional doctors will tell you that type 1 diabetes is incurable. We don't know of anyone who has been completely "cured" of type 1 diabetes other than those lucky enough to get a pancreas transplant. It is well established that improved blood sugar control can prevent some of those terrible side effects, but there are many things that Korean ginseng can do to improve the disease and lessen the side effects.

About 1.25 million Americans are living with type 1 diabetes.

People with the disease are four times more likely to die of any cause than the general population and seven times more likely to die of heart disease than non-diabetics. Type 1 diabetes shortens life expectancies by 11 years in men and 13 years in women.

Here's how red ginseng can help:

Korean animal studies showed that mice with type 1 diabetes not only reduced their blood sugars with *Panax ginseng*, the disease's destruction of existing insulin-producing islet cells was stopped, and production of the pancreas's natural insulin was increased. The study published in 2012 in the *Journal of Ethnopharmacology* also confirmed that Korean ginseng enhanced immune function as part of its anti-diabetic effects.

Taiwanese researchers found that the Rh2 ginsenoside slowed the progression of cardiac fibrosis, the thickening of the heart valves that is part of heart failure that frequently accompanies type 1 diabetes.

GINSENG AND TYPE 2

People with Type 2 diabetes are able to produce insulin just fine, but their bodies are unable to use it efficiently, and maybe not at all in the later stages.

Insulin is a hormone. That means it is a chemical messenger that sends messages to the muscles, body fat and liver to grab glucose out of the bloodstream and deposit in cells where it can be used for energy. Sugar builds up in the bloodstream, causing diabetes.

The vast majority of people with type 2 diabetes—about 90%—are overweight. And about 30% of all obese people have diabetes. Recent Harvard research concluded that overeating causes stress to cell membranes and eventually turns off the cells' components that accept insulin, causing insulin resistance.

Inflammation is part of the complicated formula that creates diabetes, so red ginseng's anti-inflammatory properties are part of its power against the disease. Free radical oxidation is another component of diabetes, calling on another of the herb's most important healing powers.

Oxidative stress and inflammation lead to the formation of AGEs-advanced glycation end products—that quite literally age the body and contribute to the heart complications that go hand-in-hand with type 2 diabetes

People with type 2 diabetes depend on a variety of oral medications and sometimes insulin injections, too. Type 2 diabetes was at one time called "adult-onset diabetes," affecting most of its victims in late middle age. In the past 20 years, when childhood obesity became epidemic, children as young as 3 (yes, 3!) have been diagnosed with the disease. Type 2 diabetes has become distressingly common in teenagers.

Worse yet are the side effects of type 2 diabetes, including heart disease and stroke, Alzheimer's, peripheral neuropathy and circulatory problems that can necessitate amputations, blindness and kidney failure, just to name a few.

Even when type 2 diabetes is treated, poor blood sugar control can damage organs, causing complications. Most early stage cases are treated with medication, diet, and exercise, while more severe cases require insulin injections.

Type 2 diabetes is one of the most prevalent diseases in the world. The American Diabetes Association estimates that 30.3 million Americans (9.4% of the population) have type 2 diabetes, and about 7.2 million of them don't know they have the disease. It is the 7th leading cause of death in the US, killing nearly 80,000 Americans a year and listed as an underlying cause of death of more than 250,000.

It's estimated that one-third of Americans will develop diabetes in their lifetimes. Diabetes should be prevented whenever possible and blood sugars should be controlled to prevent the severe side effects.

Conventional medicine has recently identified a condition called "pre-diabetes," which means that a person has elevated blood sugars that have not yet progressed to full-blown type 2 diabetes. This is often associated with high blood pressure, and elevated cholesterol—a triad called metabolic syndrome. Research suggests that ginseng can help all three of these. *Panax ginseng* has also been scientifically validated as an excellent way to prevent diabetes, along with proper diet and exercise.

HERE'S SOME OF THE MOST IMPORTANT RESEARCH ON RED GINSENG AND DIABETES:

- Numerous studies show that it is an antioxidant and anti-inflammatory, making it an effective tool for healing all sorts of illnesses, including both types of diabetes.
- A large Chinese review of existing literature, published in the journal *Cells* in 2019,

concluded that the Rb1 ginsenoside improves insulin resistance, addressing most aspects of type 2 diabetes.

- A wide-ranging Chinese study published in 2018 in *Frontiers in Pharmacology* proclaims ginseng and a plethora of ginsenosides as effective treatment for diabetes, also addressing nearly every side effect, including kidney failure, heart attack, stroke, cognitive dysfunction (dementia) and much more, highlighting Rg1, Rg3, Rb1, and Compound K as the ginsenosides most effective in addressing the myriad issues of both types of diabetes.
- Red ginseng also has been shown to reduce cardiovascular symptoms in people with type 2 diabetes, effectively addressing heart disease, one of the most life-threatening side effects of the disease.
- Two ginsenosides in red ginseng seem to attack fat cells, reducing obesity and minimizing the risk of type 2 diabetes, according to a 2017 Korean study.

WHAT YOU NEED TO KNOW:

- There are two basic types of diabetes: type 1 is a failure of the pancreas to produce sufficient insulin to balance blood sugars and type 2 is a failure of the body to utilize the insulin the pancreas produces to balance sugars.
- Both types of diabetes can lead to serious and sometimes fatal side effects, so it is important to prevent the disease from taking hold or, if it is already present, from progressing.
- Four particular ginsenosides in red ginseng have been scientifically validated as effective means of treating type 1 and type 2 diabetes and preventing some of the extremely serious side effects of both diseases.
- It combats inflammation and acts as an antioxidant, addressing some of the most important underlying causes of both types of diabetes.
- It is also shown to lower blood sugars, prevent insulin resistance and address obesity, the major cause of type 2 diabetes.

CHAPTER 7
Erectile Dysfunction Relief

Here's some important info for our male readers and their partners.

Erectile dysfunction—two little words that can make even the most macho man's knees go weak. At the very least, when the conversation turns to topics below the belt, most men become noticeably uncomfortable.

Yet, even though it's the most common male reproductive disease in the United States, less than 25% of men with erectile dysfunction seek treatment, perhaps because they are embarrassed.

Those who do visit their doctors often walk out with a prescription for sildenafil (Viagra) or tadalafil (Cialis). Yet, despite the pharmaceutical industry's prediction of "better loving through chemistry," those trendy prescriptions aren't a cure-all and can have major side effects.

Fortunately, there are natural alternatives that can safely enhance your performance and boost your zest for life with no side effects.

YOU'RE NOT ALONE!

If you are having a performance malfunction in the bedroom, you're not alone! Erectile dysfunction (ED) affects an estimated 20 to 30 million American men at some point in their lives. In fact, mild to moderate ED affects approximately 10% of men per decade of life. For instance, according to the Massachusetts Male Aging Study, 40% of men in their 40s suffer from ED and nearly 70% are affected by age 70.

While age seems to be the strongest factor for developing ED, there's a worrisome trend that was reported in 2013 in the *Journal of Sexual Medicine,* which found that one in four men seeking help for ED was under the age of 40! Plus, nearly half of the men surveyed suffered from a severe case of the condition, compared to just 40% of men over the age of 40. This puts a new face to findings from an early study—the National Health and Social Life Survey—which found that sexual dysfunction was more likely among men in poor physical and emotional health, regardless of age.

Diabetes and the circulatory disorders that often accompany Type 2 diabetes can also be a contributing factor in erectile dysfunction. At least one study shows that men with diabetes are three times as likely to have ED than men of their own age who do not have diabetes.

It sounds like a dire picture, but there is plenty you can do to prevent becoming one of these statistics at any age. And it starts here.

ANATOMY OF AN ERECTION

To really grasp the cause of ED, you first need to understand what happens inside your body when things go right. If you think of an erection like a hydraulic event, you're right—but the mechanics of the penis are only half the equation. An erection is the result of a delicate but perfectly balanced process that involves the brain, blood vessels, nerves, and hormones. If just one of those elements isn't functioning, ED can be the result.

To simplify this intricate process, let's compare an erection to a rocket launch. Here's how it works: Think of the brain as the mission control center for erections. Once mission control receives data—an erotic fantasy, a seductive photograph, even a particular scent—it sends tiny messengers called neurotransmitters to the launch pad, better known as the penile nerves. This reflex action is helped along by testosterone, the male hormone.

After the penile nerves have been aroused, other neurotransmitters trigger the release of nitric oxide (NO). This, in turn, increases blood flow to the penile arteries, causing them to expand. As the penile tissue grows in width and length, the excess blood is trapped, causing the penis to become hard and erect. In other words, Houston, we have lift off!

But when you have ED, it doesn't always work out that way.

WHY ME?

As complex as this process is, it's a wonder that things don't go awry more often. When they do go wrong, it can send a man into an emotional tailspin. Perhaps this is why, until recently, most doctors thought that ED was primarily caused by psychological factors. And, while fatigue, stress, or the uncertainties of a new relationship can cause a temporary loss of erectile function, medical science now estimates that between 80 and 90% of ED cases are caused by underlying medical problems and lifestyle factors.

COMMON RISK FACTORS FOR ED

MEDICAL	LIFESTYLE
Atherosclerosis	Alcohol Overindulgence
Benign Prostatic Hyperplasia	Anxiety
Certain Prescription Medications	Chronic Stress
Depression	Depression
Diabetes	Diet Full of Processed/ Fast Food
High Blood Pressure	Fatigue
Kidney Disease	Lack of Exercise
Low Testosterone Levels	Overweight or Obesity

MEDICAL	LIFESTYLE
Multiple Sclerosis	Poor Communication with Partner
Neurological Diseases	Recreational Drugs
Peyronie's Disease	Sedentary Lifestyle
Radiation Therapy	Smoking
Spinal Cord Injury	Stroke

But taking a proactive approach can help reduce the risk of ED. Eat smart, ditch those bad behaviors you picked up in college, and see your doctor at least once a year to make sure your blood sugar and blood pressure are okay. Not only will this help you perform at your best in the short-term, you'll be healthy and vibrant for many years to come.

THE CARDIOVASCULAR CONNECTION

ED can definitely cause heartache—in more ways than one! In fact, ED can be an early warning sign of hidden heart disease. According to an Australian study that appeared in the journal *PLoS Medicine*, even men with a mild case of ED and no known heart issues face a major risk of developing cardiovascular problems. And as ED worsens, so does the risk.

During the study of 95,000 men, age 45 and up with no signs of heart disease, those with moderate to severe ED were 50% more likely to be hospitalized for cardiovascular problems than men without ED. While having ED isn't an automatic ticket to the cardiac unit at your local hospital, if you are having problems in the bedroom, it's wise to check with your doctor.

If you've been diagnosed with ED, you might think that your options are limited to prescription drugs, hormone therapy or mechanical erectile aids. Fortunately, nothing could be further from the truth. Modern science has found that red ginseng, an ancient remedy that is a safe, natural and effective alternative to pharmaceuticals and devices, can enhance both your performance and your energy, in and out of the bedroom.

Red ginseng has a long history as an aphrodisiac and has been used for centuries in Traditional Chinese Medicine to treat sexual dysfunction, low libido, and infertility.

We already know that those magical rare ginsenosides protect against oxidative stress, so in this case, they can overcome oxidative stress in the blood vessels and penile tissue to help restore normal function. Ginsenosides in Panax ginseng increase blood circulation by promoting the production of nitrous oxide, or NO, boosting blood flow throughout the body, including to the penis.

SCIENCE SAYS . . .

Because of these actions, a growing number of studies are pointing to Panax ginseng as a safe and effective alternative to pharmaceuticals. During one double-blind, placebo-controlled clinical trial of 60 men with mild to moderate ED, more than 66% of those taking red ginseng reported improved erection. Those in the ginseng group also experienced greater rigidity, more effective penetration, and more ease maintaining their erection compared to the men in the placebo group. This study appeared in the *Asian Journal of Andrology*.

Another study in the Journal of Urology found similar results. Among the 45 participants taking part in this trial, 60% of those taking Panax ginseng scored significantly higher on the *International Index of Erectile Function* than those taking a placebo. These men reported a notable improvement in penile tip rigidity, improved erection, penetration and maintenance of erections.

An additional investigation of 86 men with ED published in the *Asian Journal of Andrology*, found that those who were treated with Panax ginseng for eight weeks had marked improvement in their erections. The men also reported an uptick in overall sexual satisfaction. The men taking a placebo, however, didn't experience any of these benefits. The researchers in this particular study credit ginsenosides for this improvement in ability and performance.

A recent study of the structural-activity relationship of ginsenosides shows that rare ginsenosides, Rg5 and Rk1, are the most effective in improving erection by lowering calcium concentration in the cells, relaxing the muscles surrounding the arteries. This way, more blood can enter the penis, resulting in an erection. At the same time, the veins are compressed, trapping the blood in the penis, sustaining the erection.

Dopamine, a neurotransmitter in the brain that gives a feeling of pleasure, plays a key role in sexual behavior. Rg3 blocks the re-uptake of dopamine which increases its synaptic availability and leads to more pleasure.

WHAT YOU NEED TO KNOW:

- Erectile dysfunction is common, especially as a man ages.
- Commonly prescribed pharmaceuticals to address erectile dysfunction (ED) such as Viagra and Cialis can have serious side effects.
- Red ginseng safely and naturally improves erectile function by optimizing blood flow when specific ginsenosides enhance the production of nitrous oxide.

CHAPTER 8
And a Grab Bag of Ailments

Ginseng has been used to address a variety of health conditions for millennia. The human-shaped root may foretell red ginseng's effectiveness in treating a broad range of conditions, some with obvious linkages to combating inflammation or neutralizing free radicals. Other effects are mysterious, but science is validating them.

Let's take a look at a few:

MENOPAUSE

It may surprise you to know that women's hormones can fluctuate wildly throughout their lives and even more so after menopause.

The adaptogenic properties of *Panax ginseng* provide relief for the symptoms associated with estrogen fluctuation during perimenopause (the years before the complete cessation of menstruation) and menopause, when the ovaries stop producing estrogen.

The results of stabilizing estrogen levels can be enormous, according to a 2018 Chinese study that showed red ginseng's far-ranging effects on menopausal animals that included promoting weight loss and stabilizing levels of two key hormones: serum luteinizing hormone, produced by the pituitary gland that opposes and balances estrogen, and serum estradiol, the female hormone produced in the ovaries, but also in the adrenal glands and liver, that is often used in hormone therapy for menopausal women.

Other studies confirm that red ginseng helps relieve the hot flashes and night sweats, mood swings and depression that often accompany menopause. It has also been shown to help prevent bone loss.

Menopause often results in lower sex drive. We've already investigated the herb's ability to relieve and even reverse erectile dysfunction. Now Korean research shows that the Korean wonder herb increases sexual arousal in menopausal women as well.

WEIGHT LOSS

While weight gain is often associated with menopause, we all know that excess weight is common in Americans at any age. In fact, over half of all-American adults are overweight. Any way to address this national problem is most welcome!

Red ginseng to the rescue!

Lab and animal studies credit ginsenosides with increasing metabolism, meaning they help you burn calories faster and curb your appetite so fewer calories are consumed.

One particular ginsenoside, Rb2, has been proven to increase insulin sensitivity in animals with Type 2 diabetes *and* to reduce body weight, largely by boosting metabolism, according to Chinese research.

Although *Panax ginseng* has been used historically for weight loss in Traditional Chinese Medicine, modern science hasn't caught up yet with human studies to validate the findings of those lab and animal studies.

HEART DISEASE

Heart disease falls in the same category as type 2 diabetes, various types of arthritis, some types of cancer and Alzheimer's disease, because inflammation is an underlying cause of them all.

As we've mentioned, red ginseng is a power anti-inflammatory, so by its very nature, this Asian herb addresses these diseases—including heart disease—at their roots. Among the many properties attributed to 40 unique ginsenosides, a 2012 Korean review of existing studies shows that Korean ginseng reduces blood pressure and blood fats, including cholesterol.

IMMUNE SYSTEM BOOSTER

Short-term use of Korean ginseng when symptoms of colds and flu arise is effective because it helps boost immune function.

Some studies suggest using red ginseng as a preventive during the winters and show it may shorten the duration of a viral illness if you get one.

Korean researchers also found that red ginseng enhances the effectiveness of the pneumonia vaccine.

LUNG FUNCTION

Beyond its effectiveness against pneumonia and other respiratory attacks, Korean ginseng helps reduce bacteria in the lungs and has been traditionally used to improve breathing in patients with conditions like chronic obstructive pulmonary disease (COPD). Research on this effect is still in the early stages.

HEPATITIS C

Solid research shows that Korean ginseng kills the hepatitis C virus, a deadly liver disease for which there is no vaccine. There is a treatment/cure with a drug called interferon, but its administration and side effects are brutal.

The Rg3 ginsenoside is a known liver protectant, but new research goes a lot farther. Korean research published in the journal *Hepatology* in 2017 concluded that Rg3 attacks the hepatitis C virus and suppresses chronic infection.

HANGOVER

If you've overindulged, red ginseng can come to the rescue. It helps ease morning-after pain in the brain by increasing the enzymes that help in alcohol breakdown. According to a study performed at the Teaching Hospital of Chengdu University of Traditional Chinese Medicine, it has positive effects on acute alcohol intoxication.

Plus, researchers concluded, the antioxidant activity of *Panax ginseng* helped protect against long-term digestive and reproductive problems.

CHAPTER 9
What You Need to Know

From Terry Lemerond:

So what exactly are these magical performance-boosting ginsenosides and how can you choose the right product to maximize your results?

Panax ginseng contains more than 50 different ginsenosides, which, as you already know, are responsible for its main medicinal benefits. However, the vast majority of ginsenosides aren't absorbed well by the body.

Ginsenosides are protective plant compounds produced by red ginseng in response to stressors like predators (mainly insects) or extreme climate changes. They work to protect you and promote good health, too.

To be effective, those ginsenosides must be converted to what science calls "rare" ginsenosides by the beneficial bacteria in your gut. Once this happens, these rare ginsenosides are more easily absorbed and more available for your body to use (bioavailable) than the original ginsenosides. Unfortunately, however, much is usually lost during this conversion process.

It's important to remember that red ginseng also contains a treasure house of other health-producing nutrients, including:

- Polyacetylenes such as panaxynol known to target cancer stem cells and kill those undying cancer cells
- Polyphenolic compounds, powerful antioxidants that target all of the diseases of aging
- Arginine and its derivatives that produce nitric oxide, helping widen blood vessels and stimulate the release of insulin and human growth hormone.
- Acidic polysaccharides that play a key role in digestion and energy production.

This all adds up to an impressive array of ingredients for optimal health.

Not-so-clean ginseng

But there a catch. Isn't there always?

While ginseng has been cultivated for medicinal use for centuries, modern agricultural practices—including heavy pesticide and fungicide spraying as well as processing with toxic chemicals—have undercut the herb's effectiveness and safety.

As a result, it's been increasingly difficult to find ethically grown and responsibly processed ginseng with enhanced absorption and bioavailability.

Most red ginseng used in supplements is teased out of the root using harsh solvents. The problem is this method can only extract a fraction of the active beneficial molecules and bioactive ingredients.

What's missing? Fiber, protein and a host of minerals and vitamins that provide added health benefits.

Of more concern, solvent extraction can hide adulterations—things like the inclusion of leaves or other parts of the plant, or even other species like Panax quinquefolius (also known as American ginseng, a helpful herb that has very different health benefits). Solvents can also hide poor quality or irradiated ginseng or pesticide contamination. Some products that are processed this way can even carry solvent residue that can be harmful to your health!

A SAFE WAY

There's an answer to all of those "catches" that ticks all the boxes for safety and effectiveness.

The method of producing the red ginseng HRG80™ formulation begins with plants grown hydroponically in Belgium. There are no pesticides, insecticides or GMOs used in the growing process, meaning this clean product is now available to us all.

After harvest, the roots are processed without the use of any solvents, using traditional Korean steam cooking and drying to extract the nutrients.

This method not only concentrates the rare ginsenosides and other valuable nutrients, it also pro-duces an ultra-pure and environmentally responsible ginseng supplement that is, in my opinion, the most bioactive ginseng on the market. Rich in rare ginsenosides, with a potency seven times higher than any other Panax ginseng formulation, it offers better bioavailability and unprecedented effectiveness.

HOW TO FIND THE RIGHT STUFF

If you walk into any health food store to purchase your ginseng, you're likely to find some products labeled American ginseng, some labeled as Panax ginseng (sometimes called Korean white ginseng), and still others labeled as Korean red ginseng.

Confusing? You bet!

Here's the breakdown:

What about white ginseng and Korean red ginseng? They come from the same plant! The difference between the two comes from the way they are processed.

As you learned earlier, *Panax ginseng*, also known as Korean or red ginseng, sometimes as Asian ginseng, is processed using traditional methods that include steam cooking the root to its characteristic red color and then air drying it.

White ginseng, on the other hand, is dried immediately after it is harvested and peeled.

This difference in processing is what gives each its unique health properties. That's why it's important to pay attention to the color of your ginseng, especially if you suffer from fatigue and mental stress or erectile dysfunction.

American ginseng comes from a totally different species of ginseng called *Panax quinquefolius.*

To ensure you're getting a clean *Panax ginseng* product, check the front label for the words "whole root," "full spectrum," and "solvent-free." This will also ensure you are getting a supplement that doesn't contain pesticide or solvent residue or mold toxins.

WHAT YOU NEED TO KNOW:

- Many *Panax ginseng* products are mass produced, adulterated with pesticides and herbicides.
- They are processed using harmful solvents.
- All of these adulterants can end up in their products.
- Hydroponic red ginseng is produced in an environmentally responsible manner without pesticides or insecticides.
- It is processed using traditional Korean steam cooking and drying methods that make it safe, clean and effective.
- The clean production process concentrates rare ginsenosides, making it by far the most effective red ginseng formulation available.

CHAPTER 10
DOC TO DOC: What the Science Says About Ginseng

From Dr. Teitelbaum:

Dear Doctor,

Thank you for agreeing to spend a few minutes increasing your knowledge of *Panax ginseng*, one of the most important ingredients in today's natural medicine chest and an excellent natural treatment option for your patients.

First, allow me to introduce myself: I'm Jacob Teitelbaum, M.D., a practitioner of integrative medicine and author of numerous books, including one I wrote many years ago called From Fatigued to Fantastic (now in its fourth edition). I've spent much of my career investigating human fatigue and energy, and finding natural ways to address both, producing measurable benefits for my patients.

Panax ginseng, also known as red ginseng, Korean ginseng or Asian ginseng, has been used medicinally for millennia. Modern science is finally catching up with the preventive and curative properties that practitioners of Traditional Chinese Medicine and Ayurveda have long known and used.

Ginseng contains a wealth of nutrient compounds. The most important are more than 50 forms of ginsenosides, also known as steroid-like saponins. When processed in a very specific manner, these ginsenosides are transformed into "rare" ginsenosides that defend the plant from stressors, especially insects and fluctuating temperatures, thereby increasing their potency. Current scientific literature validates these rare ginsenosides as:

- Adaptogenic
- Anti-inflammatory
- Antioxidant
- Anticancer
- Antitumor
- Apoptotic
- Antidiabetic
- Anti-stress (physiological and psychological)

Plus there is a multitude of other beneficial nutrients in ginseng, including gintonins, phenols, polysaccharides, lignans, amino acids, minerals and more, each with its unique contribution to the healing powers of ginseng.

Being mindful of your time, let me give you a synopsis of the most cogent research on Panax ginseng:

FATIGUE

Panax ginseng has been shown to relieve chronic fatigue. Research published in 2007 confirms that it actually helps reduce levels of cortisol when lab animals were subjected to stressful situations. Other studies show that it helps balance the hypothalamic-pituitary-adrenal axis dysfunction. This means ginseng taken daily can halt the stress cycle and excess cortisol.

A growing number of studies point to red ginseng as a safe and effective way to reduce mental and physical fatigue and restore vitality.

MENTAL ACUITY AND COGNITIVE FUNCTION

The ginsenoside metabolite Compound K, an antioxidant biotransformed from ginsenosides Rb1, Rb2 and Rc, has been shown to improve memory and protect the brain from age-related cognitive decline, and decrease the effects of Alzheimer's disease and cerebral ischemia.

The authors of a Korean study concluded, "The plethora of potential health benefits of Compound K war-rants further research to evaluate its biochemical mechanisms and its ability to protect healthy populations from neurodegenerative diseases."

In my opinion, the results are significant enough to use Panax ginseng for the prevention of neurodegenerative disease given that there are no serious negative side effects.

TYPE 1 DIABETES MITIGATION

Korean animal studies showed that mice with type 1 diabetes not only reduced their blood sugars with red ginseng, the disease's destruction of existing insulin-producing islet cells was stopped, and production of the pancreas's natural insulin was increased. The study published in 2012 in the *Journal of Ethnopharmacology* also confirmed that Korean ginseng enhanced immune function as part of its anti-diabetic effects.

Taiwanese researchers found that the Rh2 ginsenoside slowed the progression of cardiac fibrosis.

TYPE 2 DIABETES MITIGATION

A large Chinese review of existing literature, published in the journal *Cells* in 2019, concluded that the Rb1 ginsenoside improves insulin resistance, addressing most aspects of type 2 diabetes.

A wide-ranging Chinese study published in 2018 in *Frontiers in Pharmacology* proclaims ginseng and a plethora of ginsenosides as effective treatment for virtually all types of diabetes and addressing nearly every side effect, including kidney failure, heart attack, stroke, cognitive dysfunction (dementia) and much more, high-lighting Rg1, Rg3, Rb1, and Compound K as the ginsenosides most effective in addressing the myriad issues of both types of diabetes.

Panax ginseng also has been shown to reduce cardiovascular symptoms in people with type 2 diabetes, effectively addressing one of the most life-threatening side effects of the disease.

A number of studies show that it also has promise for helping all the components of metabolic syndrome. Two ginsenosides in Panax ginseng also appear to impact adipocytes, reducing obesity and minimizing the risk of diabetes, according to a 2017 Korean study.

CANCER

Dozens of studies suggest that red ginseng is a powerful tool in cancer prevention and treatment when processed using the traditional steaming method.

Red ginseng is credited with approaching cancer in four ways: cell cycle arrest, inducing apoptosis, curbing angiogenesis, and as an anti-metastatic. It is also a preventive and a chemo-enhancer and its anti-inflammatory effects are an important preventive tool especially for those at high risk for cancer.

Researchers in a 2001 Korean study concluded, "... Panax ginseng has been established as non-organ specific preventive, having dose response relationship. These results warrant that ginseng extracts and its synthetic derivatives should be examined for their preventive effect on various types of human cancers." Research has shown that it even significantly improves cancer-related fatigue.

ERECTILE DYSFUNCTION

Red ginseng is a safe, natural and effective alternative to pharmaceuticals and devices.

Ginsenosides increase blood circulation by promoting the production of nitric oxide. A growing number of studies confirm its effect on erectile dysfunction.

A study in the *Journal of Urology* found similar results. Among the 45 participants taking part in this trial, 60% of those taking Korean red ginseng scored significantly higher on the *International Index of Erectile Function* than those taking a placebo. These men reported a notable improvement in penile tip rigidity, improved erection, penetration, and maintenance.

An additional investigation of 86 men with ED published in the *Asian Journal of Andrology,* found that those who were treated with red ginseng for eight weeks had marked improvement in the quality of their erections. The men also reported an uptick in overall sexual satisfaction. The placebo group didn't experience any of these benefits. The researchers in this particular study credit rare ginsenosides for this improvement in ability and performance.

Additional beneficial effects

MENOPAUSAL SYMPTOMS

Red ginseng has been shown to be effective in stabilizing estrogen and luteinizing hormone levels in menopausal women, increasing libido, moderating hot flashes, night sweats, depression and mood swings typical of perimenopause and menopause and improving sexual function in menopausal women.

WEIGHT LOSS

Lab and animal studies credit ginsenosides with increasing metabolism and one particular ginsenoside, Rb2, has been proven to increase insulin sensitivity in animals with type 2 diabetes and to reduce body weight, largely by boosting metabolism, according to Chinese research.

LUNG FUNCTION

Beyond its effectiveness against pneumonia and other respiratory diseases, Panax ginseng helps reduce bacteria in the lungs and has been traditionally used to improve breathing in patients with conditions like chronic obstructive pulmonary disease. Research on this effect is still in the early stages.

HEPATITIS C

Solid research shows that Panax ginseng kills the hepatitis C virus.

Korean research published in the journal *Hepatology* in 2017 concluded that Rg3 attacks the hepatitis C virus and suppresses chronic infection.

HANGOVER

Red ginseng helps ease morning-after pain in the brain by increasing the enzymes that help in alcohol breakdown. According to a study performed at the Teaching Hospital of Chengdu University of Traditional Chinese Medicine in China, it has positive effects on acute alcohol intoxication. Additionally, the antioxidant activity of Panax ginseng helped protect against long-term digestive and reproductive problems.

PRODUCT SPECIFICS

Until very recently, Panax ginseng has had limited bioavailability. A new hydroponic production method, coupled with traditional Korean steam processing has been validated with enhanced bioavailability, largely through dramatically increased production of rare ginsenosides.

This is my choice for efficacy and bioavailability. Assays validate it is 17 times more bioavailable, and it has seven times more rare ginsenosides than standard ginseng preparations.

I highly recommend this formulation to you and your patients.

—Jacob Teitelbaum MD

References

Chapter 1: A Prized Herbal Remedy

Choi J. Ginseng for health care: a systematic review of randomized controlled trials in Korean literature. *PLoS One*. 2013;8(4):e59978.

He M, Huang X. The Difference between White and Red Ginseng: Variations in Ginsenosides and Immunomodulation. *Planta Med.* 2018 Aug;84(12-13):845-854. doi: 10.1055/a-0641-6240. Epub 2018 Jun 20.

Kim HJ. Panax ginseng as an adjuvant treatment for Alzheimer's disease. *J Ginseng Res.* 2018;42(4):401-11.

Chi H, Ji GE. Transformation of ginsenosides Rb1 and Re from Panax ginseng by food microorganisms. *Biotechnol Lett.* 2005; 27:765–71.

Wai-Nam Sung, Hoi-Hin Jwok, Man-Hee Rhee et al. Korean Red Ginseng extract induces angiogenesis through activation of glucocorticoid receptor. *J Ginseng Res.* 2017 Oct; 41(4): 477–486.

Pan W. Biopharmaceutical characters and bioavailability improving strategies of ginsenosides. *Fitoterapia.* 2018;129:272-82.

Chapter 2: The Great Multi-Tasker

Scaglione F. Efficacy and safety of the standardized ginseng extract G115 for potentiating vaccination against the influenza syndrome and protection against the common cold. *Drugs Exp Clin Res.* 1996;22(2):65-72.

Kim JH. Role of ginsenosides, the main active components of *Panax ginseng*, in inflammatory responses and diseases. *J Ginseng Res.* 2016;41(4):435-443.

Yu S, Zhou X, Li F, Xu C, Zheng F, Li J, Zhao H, Dai Y, Liu S, Feng Y. Microbial transformation of ginsenoside Rb1, Re and Rg1 and its contribution to the improved anti-inflammatory activity of ginseng. Sci Rep. 2017 Mar 10;7(1):138.

Lee YM, Yoon H et al. Implications of red *Panax ginseng* in oxidative stress associated chronic diseases. *J Ginseng Res.* 2017 Apr; 41(2): 113–119.

Chapter 3: Where's My Get Up and Go?

Arring NM. Ginseng as a treatment for fatigue: A systematic review. *Altern Complement Med.* 2018;24(7):624-633.

Baek JH. Effect of Korean red ginseng in individuals exposed to high stress levels: a 6-week, double-blind, randomized, placebo-controlled trial. J Ginseng Res. 2018:1-6.

Bach HV. Efficacy of ginseng supplements on fatigue and physical performance: a meta-analysis. J Korean Med Sci. 2016;31(12):1879-86.

Kim JH. Antifatigue effects of Panax ginseng C.A. Meyer: a randomized, double-blind, placebo-controlled trial. PLoS One. 2013;8(4):e61271.

Kaneko H. Proof of the mysterious efficacy of ginseng: basic and clinical trials: clinical effects of medical ginseng, Korean red ginseng: specifically, its anti-stress action for prevention of disease. *J Pharmacol Sci.* 2004;95(2):158-62.

Chapter 4: A Better Brain

Radad K. Use of ginseng in medicine with emphasis on neurodegenerative disorders. *J Pharmacol Sci.* 2006 Mar;100(3):175-86.

Kim HJ. Panax ginseng as an adjuvant treatment for Alzheimer's disease. *J Ginseng Res.* 2018;42(4):401-11.

Yeo HB. Effects of Korean red ginseng on cognitive and motor function: A double-blind, randomized, placebo-controlled trial. *J Ginseng Res.* 2012;36(2):190-7.

Chi H, Ji GE. Transformation of ginsenosides Rb1 and Re from Panax ginseng by food microorganisms. Biotechnol Lett. 2005; 27:765–71.

Cooley K. Naturopathic care for anxiety: a randomized controlled trial ISRCTN78958974. *PLoS One.* 2009;4(8):e6628.

Chapter 5: Cancer Combatant

Wang CZ, Anderson DU WS et al. Red ginseng and cancer treatment. *Chin J Nat Med.* 2016 Jan;14(1):7-16. doi: 10.3724/SP.J.1009.2016.00007.

Chen XJ, X.J. Zhang XJ, Y.M. ShuiYM, et al., Anticancer activities of protopanaxadioland protopanaxatriol-type ginsenosides and their metabolites, Evid. Based Complement. *Alternat. Med.* 2016 (4) (2016) 1–19.

Oh M, Choi YH, Choi S, Chung H, Kim K. Anti-proliferating effects of ginsenoside Rh2 on MCF-7 human breast cancer cells. *Int J Oncol* 1999;14:869e75.

Mai TT, Moon JY, Song YW. Ginsenoside F2 induces apoptosis accompanied by protective autophagy in breast cancer stem cells. *Cancer Lett* 2012;321: 144e53.

Yue PY, Mak NK, Cheng YK, Leung KW, Ng TB, Fan DT, Yeung HW, Wong RN. Pharmacogenomics and the Yin/ Yang actions of ginseng: anti-tumor, angiomodulating and steroid-like activities of ginsenosides. *Chin Med.* 2007 May 15;2:6.

Seo EY, Kim, WK. nRed Ginseng Extract Reduced Metastasis of Colon Cancer Cells *In Vitro* and *In Vivo. J Ginseng Res.* 2011 Sep; 35(3): 315–324.

Chapter 6: Diabetes—Two Types—and Better Control

Bang H. Korean red ginseng improves glucose control in subjects with impaired fasting glucose, impaired glucose tolerance, or newly diagnosed type 2 diabetes mellitus. *J Med Food.* 2014;17(1):128-34.

Hong YI, Kim N et al. Korean red ginseng (Panax ginseng) ameliorates type 1 diabetes and restores immune cell compartments. *Int J Mol Sci.* 2017 Jun 26;18(7).

Mairino MI, Bellastrella G, Espositio K. Diabetes and sexual dysfunction: current perspectives. *Diabetes Metab Syndr Obes.* 2014; 7: 95–105.

Zhou P. Ginsenoside Rb1 as an Anti-Diabetic Agent and Its Underlying Mechanism Analysis. *Cells.* 2019 Feb 28;8(3).

Chapter 7: Erectile Dysfunction Relief

Choi HK. Clinical efficacy of Korean red ginseng for erectile dysfunction. *Int J Impot Res.* 1995;7(3):181-6.

Li H. Panax notoginseng saponins improve erectile function through attenuation of oxidative stress, restoration of Akt activity and protection of endothelial and smooth muscle cells in diabetic rats with erectile dysfunction. *Urol Int.* 2014;93(1):92-9.

Jang DJ. Red ginseng for treating erectile dysfunction: a systematic review. *Br J Clin Pharmacol.* 2008;66(4):444-50

Kim TH. Effects of tissue-cultured mountain ginseng *Panax ginseng* CA Meyer) extract on male patients with erectile dysfunction. *Asian J Androl.* 2009;11(3):356-61.

Chapter 8: And a Grab Bag of Other Ailments

Kim SY. Effects of red ginseng supplementation on menopausal symptoms and cardiovascular risk factors in postmenopausal women: A double-blind randomized controlled trial. *Menopause.* 2012;19(4):461-6.

Lee HW. Ginseng for managing menopausal women's health: A systematic review of double-blind, randomized, placebo-controlled trials. *Medicine (Baltimore).* 2016;95(38):e4914.

Oh KJ, Chae Mj et al. Effects of Korean red ginseng on sexual arousal in menopausal women: placebo-controlled, double-blind crossover clinical study. *J Sex Med.* 2010 Apr;7(4 Pt 1):1469-77.

Siraj FM, SathishKumar N, Kim YJ. Ginsenoside F2 possesses anti-obesity activity via binding with PPAR and inhibiting adipocyte differentiation in the 3T3-L1 cell line. *J Enzym Inhib Med* Ch 2014;30:9e14.

Wang F, Li Y, Zhang YL. Natural Products for the Prevention and Treatment of Hangover and Alcohol Use Disorder. *Molecules.* 2016 Jan; 21(1): 64.

About the Authors

Terry Lemerond

Terry Lemerond is a natural health expert with over 50 years of experience helping people live healthier, happier lives. A much sought-after speaker and accomplished author, Terry shares his wealth of experience and knowledge in health and nutrition through his educational programs, including the Terry Talks Nutrition website TerryTalksNutrition.com—newsletters, podcasts, webinars, and personal speaking engagements. Terry has also hosted Terry Talks Nutrition radio for the past 30 years.

The following books are available on Amazon in Kindle Unlimited, as eBooks, and as paperbacks:

Fight Disease With A Powerful Natural Seed–The Wonders of French Grape Seed Extract

Nature's Disease Fighter–Andrographis

Type 2 Diabetes? Break Free Naturally, with Hintonia

Wake UP! Melatonin is For More Than Just Sleep

Relieve Pain without Side Effects

Trauma Comfrey, Nature's Healing Herb

Drug-Free Relief of Anxiety & Stress

Propolis, The Natural Way to Prevent and Heal Infection

Restore Your Health with the Wise Ginseng Choice

Polyphenol Power!

The Mediterranean Anti-Aging Secret to Vibrant Health– Greek Mountain Tea is the Ancient Secret to: Improved Mental Clarity. Reduced Anxiety. Strong Immunity. Bone Density. Preventing Alzheimer's Disease

Outsmart Cancer with Powerful Natural Medicines

Reduce Fatty Liver with Herbal Medicines

Also available in paperback:

Seven Keys to Vibrant Health

Seven Keys to Unlimited Personal Achievement

50+ Natural Health Secrets Proven to Change Your Life

Discovering Your Best Health – How to Improve Your Health at Any Age

Terry continues to author and co-author books to educate everyone on the steps they can take to live a healthier, vibrant life.

His continual dedication, energy, and zeal are part of his ongoing mission—to help us all improve our health.

JACOB TEITELBAUM, M.D.

Jacob Teitelbaum, M.D., is one of the most frequently quoted integrative medical authorities in the world. He is the author of the best-selling books: *From Fatigued to Fantastic!,*

Pain Free, 1,2,3!,

The Complete Guide to Beating Sugar Addiction,

Real Cause Real Cure,

The Fatigue and Fibromyalgia Solution

And the popular, free smart phone app *Cures A–Z.*

He is the lead author of numerous research studies and appears often as a guest on news and talk shows nationwide, including *Good Morning America, The Dr. Oz Show, Oprah & Friends, CNN* and *Fox News Health.* Learn more at www.Vitality101.com.

More about TTN Publishing, LLC

Everyone has the same desire:
a vibrant, healthy life!

TTN Publishing exists to provide educational information anyone can use to understand how herbs and botanical medicines play a vital role in optimal health. From a stomachache to a life-threatening disease, even cancer, the plant kingdom has safe, effective phytonutrients and answers for healthy living.

Author and health pioneer Terry Lemerond brings his vast knowledge of plant medicines combined with cutting edge research from today's top scientists and doctors directly to consumers.

Each TTN Publishing, LLC book is crafted to provide the necessary basic information and recommendations for how botanicals can be used in practical ways to fight disease and improve the path to healthy living.

Education, information, scientific validation, and common sense are a part of every TTN Publishing endeavor. There are many books to come, so stay connected! With 80 percent of the world's population depending on plant medicines, you can join in the knowledge and wisdom available to meet your health goals.

Welcome to TTN Publishing!

We'd love to hear from you!
info@ttnpublishing.com
www.TTNPublishing.com

Would you like to be one of the first to know the latest updates on Terry's books?

- Learn more about his background and new books
- See photos, videos, and the latest news
- Listen to Terry's radio show, including archived programs on a multitude of subjects
- Sign up for a free weekly email newsletter and educational webinar notices

It's all available at TerryTalksNutrition.com

Don't forget to connect at:
www.facebook.com/TerryTalksNutrition

SHARE THIS EXCITING NEWS!

If you appreciated this book, please let others know.

- Pick up another copy and share with a friend
- Talk about it on social media
- Write a review on your blog or website
- Recommend this book to friends and family

Thank you for being a true health seeker!
TTN Publishing, LLC

Also by Terry Lemerond and available on Amazon

(Free in Kindle Unlimited and available in eBook and paperback)

Fight Disease with a Powerful, Natural Seed – The Wonders of French Grape Seed Extract
Prevent and Reverse: Cancer, Heart Disease, Diabetes, Alzheimer's & More
by Terry Lemerond and Ajay Goel M.S. Ph.D.
https://www.amazon.com/Fight-Disease-Powerful-Natural-Seed-ebook/dp/B08MB12PF9

Nature's Disease Fighter-Andrographis Protection Against: Colds, flu, & upper respiratory infections, joint pain and arthritis, diabetes, heart disease, liver disease, cancer, and much more!
by Terry Lemerond and Alexander Panossian, Ph.D.
https://www.amazon.com/NATURES-DISEASE-FIGHTER-ANDROGRAPHIS-Respiratory-ebook/dp/B0CCBWQ416

Type 2 Diabetes? Break Free Naturally with Hintonia
by Terry Lemerond and Jacob Teitelbaum, M.D.
https://www.amazon.com/Type-Diabetes-Break-Naturally-Hintonia-ebook/dp/B08ZT3TVP4

Relieve Pain Without Side Effects: You Can Be Pain-free, Naturally!
by Terry Lemerond and Jan McBarron M.D.
https://www.amazon.com/Relieve-Pain-Without-Side-Effects-ebook/dp/B091QCJW51

Wake UP! Melatonin is For More Than Just Sleep
by Terry Lemerond and a forward by Jacob Teitelbaum, M.D
https://www.amazon.com/Wake-Melatonin-More-Than-Sleep-ebook/dp/B092KZHR88

Trauma Comfrey, Nature's Healing Herb
by Terry Lemerond and Holly Lucille, ND, RN
https://www.amazon.com/Trauma-Comfrey-Natures-Healing-Herb-ebook/dp/B09JWRMCLJ

Drug-Free Relief of Anxiety & Stress
by Terry Lemerond and Dr. Lynn Wagner
https://www.amazon.com/Drug-Free-Relief-Anxiety-Stress-Stress-Induced-ebook/dp/B09JWVQV18

Propolis The Natural Way to Prevent and Heal Infection: Fights Infection Including: Bacterial, Viral, Fungal, Parasitic, and More
by Terry Lemerond
https://www.amazon.com/Propolis-Natural-Prevent-Heal-Infection/dp/1952507227

Polyphenol Power!
Polyphenols in fruit and vegetables to prevent and cure: Heart Disease, Cancer, Type 2 Diabetes, Alzheimer's and more!
by Terry Lemerond
https://www.amazon.com/POLYPHENOL-POWER-Polyphenols-vegetables-Alzheimers-ebook/dp/B0B6Q7GS9F

Outsmart Cancer with Powerful Natural Medicines
The Five Alternative Solutions to Prevent and Treat Cancer
by Terry Lemerond and Ajay Goel, Ph.D., AGAF
https://www.amazon.com/Outsmart-Cancer-POWERFUL-NATURAL-MEDICINES-ebook/dp/B0C6X7NQ5Q

The Mediterranean Anti-Aging Secret to Vibrant Health
Greek Mountain Tea is the Ancient Secret to:
Improved Mental Clarity. Reduced Anxiety. Strong Immunity. Bone Density. Preventing Alzheimer's Disease
by Terry Lemerond
https://www.amazon.com/MEDITERRANEAN-ANTI-AGING-SECRET-VIBRANT-HEALTH-ebook/dp/B0C5KFXSF6

Reduce Fatty Liver Disease with HERBAL MEDICINES
by Terry Lemerond and Dr. Lexi Loch
https://www.amazon.com/Reduce-Fatty-Disease-HERBAL-MEDICINES-ebook/dp/B0CCBT5F8T

By Terry Lemerond, also available in paperback on Amazon:

Discovering Your Best Health–HOW TO IMPROVE YOUR HEALTH AT ANY AGE

Terry Talks Nutrition 50+ Natural Health Secrets Proven to Change Your Life

Seven Keys to Vibrant Health

Seven Keys to Unlimited Personal Achievement

Made in the USA
Monee, IL
18 October 2026

66036209R00062

Made in the USA
Monee, IL
18 October 2026

66036204R10152